A Little Book
About Your Back

By
Ann McNeil
Occupational Therapist

Illustrations and layout
by
Ferrington Connection

D1232084

Thorsons

Thorsons
An Imprint of HarperCollins*Publishers*
77-85 Fulham Palace Road,
Hammersmith, London W6 8JB

The Thorsons website address is: www.thorsons.com

First published by Ann McNeil 1999
This edition published by Thorsons 2000

1 3 5 7 9 10 8 6 4 2

© Ann McNeil, 2001

Ann McNeil asserts the moral right to
be identified as the author of this work

A catalogue record of this book is available
from the British Library

ISBN 0 00 710661 0

Printed and bound in Hong Kong by Printing Express

Note from the Author

This little book is based on the principles that I have been teaching in "Back Schools" during the last ten years. It is not intended to be a book of rules. I hope you will use it to extract a few hints and some advice that might be suitable for you personally. In case of persistent pain, please consult an appropriate health practitioner.

Acknowledgements

For my family, back sufferers all !

Thanks to all of you for the advice, patience and practical help, and to the staff of the spine centre and the Hopital de la Tour, Geneva, Switzerland for their help and encouragement.

Do you spend much of your day sitting, standing, lifting or bending ?

Do you groan when you see a flight of stairs and immediately look for the lift ?

Would you rather watch TV than go for a walk ?

In a traffic jam do you get angry, grip the steering wheel tightly ? Is your jaw tense ?

Waiting in a queue are your legs straight and knees locked ?

Are you aware that at least 8 out of 10 people will suffer some back pain in their lives ?

 Would you like some practical advice on how to prevent or recover from back pain, and are you prepared to participate actively ?

If you answer yes to any of these questions, then read on !

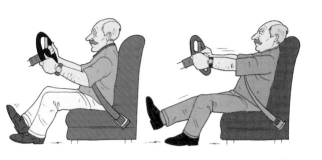

Index

	Page
Think Straight	14
Think Close	16
Think Supple	18
Keep Moving	20

Your Body, Mind and Attitude   22

- Why do so many people suffer from back or neck pain ?   22
- What can we do about it ?   23
- Where does my pain come from ?   24-27
- What to do if back pain comes on suddenly   28-29
- Your body as a whole   30
- Your teeth   31
- Your feet   32
- Your posture   34
- Stress and tension   36 & 38

- And how to cope with it   37 & 39
- Menopause and depression   40
- Male menopause   42
- Female menopause   44
- Diet   46

Activities of Daily Living   48

- The pelvic tilt   48-51
- At home: general rules   52
- Beds and bedrooms   54
- In bed   56
- Sleeping positions   58
- Your sex life   60
- The bathroom   62-65
- Shoes, socks, tights and toe nails   66
- Dress   68
- Useful positions to adopt when doing
  housework or performing heavy activities   70-71

- In the kitchen   72
- At the sink   74
- The oven or dishwasher   76
- Preparing food   78
- Shopping   80-83
- Housework: making beds   84
- Sweeping, vacuuming, cleaning the bath   86-89
- The washing machine and ironing   90-93
- Eating and at the table   94
- Armchairs and relaxing   96
- Pregnancy   98
- Babies and small children   100-103

At Work   104

- A few facts   104
- Sitting   106
- Sitting at a computer   108-111
- Chairs, seats and cushions   112

- Young people's backs, schools and studying 114-117
- Standing at work 118-121
- Standing at parties 122

Lifting and Moving 124

- A few facts 124
- Lifting light objects 126
- Pre-planned lifting of medium/ heavy objects 128
- Proper lifting of medium/ heavy objects 130
- Moving house, pushing, pulling and lifting 132
- Lifting children and adults 134-137

Transport　　　　　　　　　138

- Travelling by car　　　　　　138-141
- Packing the car and long journeys　142
- Driving lorries, vans and
  agricultural machinery　　　　144
- Travelling by plane　　　　　146
- Luggage　　　　　　　　　148

Sports and Leisure　　　150

- Introduction　　　　　　　150
- Recommended sports　　　152-159

- Sports **not** recommended　　160
- Leisure activities　　　　　162
- A word about gardening　　162

Stretching and Relaxation for the Whole Family 164

- Introduction 164
- Sitting and stretching 166-167
- Standing, lying and stretching 168-169
- Stretching for the upper back 170-171
- Stretching to **avoid** 173
- Relaxation 174

Conclusion 176

This little book offers you practical ideas about looking after your back, but your participation is needed. Write down on a large piece of paper what you think would give you less stress in your daily life. Stick it to your fridge door, or on your desk or keep it somewhere private, but somewhere you can glance at from time to time.

In order to simplify this little book, we have used colour coding throughout.

As a general guideline:

  Green and **Blue** colours are good for your back

 Red colours are not good for your back

The Four Keys to a Healthy Back

THINK STRAIGHT !

THINK CLOSE !

THINK SUPPLE !

KEEP MOVING !

THINK STRAIGHT

Try to:

- Bend with a straight back. Tighten your buttock and abdominal muscles, and bend with your knees.
- Keep straight and well balanced. Equally weighted on each side of the body.
- Walk tall.
- Maintain the natural curves of your back.

- Avoid extreme positions.
- Because we stand upright, most of our body weight rests on the vertebrae of our lower spine, the most common area of problems.
- The abdominal muscles support the back. Weak abdominals, increased weight and a protruding stomach = increased strain and pain.

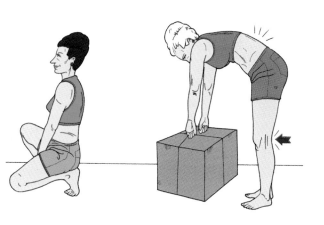

THINK CLOSE

Try to:

- Sit close to your table or desk/elbows bent and loose.
- When lifting an object bring it in close to you and use your body as a "hugging" support/elbows and knees bent.
- When searching for something in a cupboard, keep close, lean or kneel.
- If we had spent life squatting close to the ground like our ancestors, the chances are we would probably not be a generation of back sufferers.

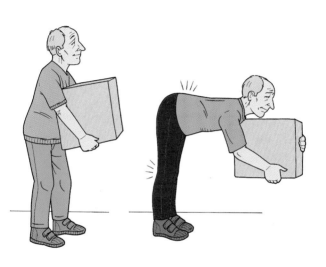

THINK SUPPLE

Try to:

- Watch a toddler moving and lifting. You did it like this once !
- Practice breathing correctly. Inhale slowly from the upper abdomen. Exhale slowly and deeply, tighten your abdomen, expel the air.
- Keep wrists, hands and fingers relaxed and flexible. Keep ankles and feet relaxed and flexible.
- Keep knees and elbows slightly bent.

- Feeling angry, depressed, tired or ill increases tension and pain.
- Tense arms and hands can cause neck and upper back pain.
- Tense legs and feet can cause lower back pain.
- The increasing demands of our lifestyle leave little time to feel relaxed.

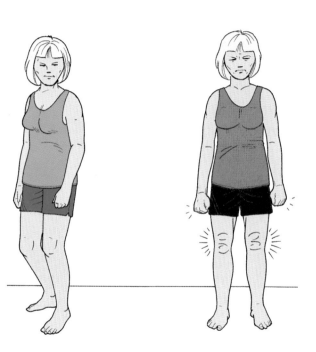

KEEP MOVING

- Our ancestors never stopped moving. They swung around trees, hunted, ran and squatted close to the ground.

- We have become a sedentary race preferring motorised transport to our own feet, preferring to relax in front of a computer or a TV and economically, millions of dollars, pounds, francs, whatever currency you like is being lost by employers or is being spent on medical help every year because people suffer from back pain, hence causing a major problem, especially in the Western world.

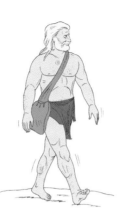

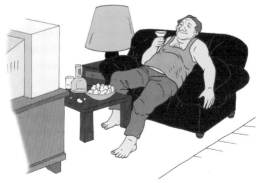

YOUR BODY, MIND AND ATTITUDE

Why do so many people suffer from back or neck pain ?

- We may have too much to do, with too little time to do it in.
- There may be too many pressures in modern life. Will I lose my job this week or next ? How can I pay all my bills ?
- We are too sedentary.
- Most furniture is made to be economically viable, not ergonomically viable.
- We are growing taller in successive generations, but heights of working surfaces have not adapted accordingly.
- We are an ageing population; will our backs take those extra years ?
- All of these factors and more accumulate to produce tension and stress.
- A tense body needs an outlet. We may have back pain, tension headaches or digestive problems.

- Because we are too busy, we ignore the first signs of what may become a long term, chronic problem.

What can we do about it ?

- Keep fit and keep walking: Did you know that 80% of back pain can be traced back to lack of exercise ?
- Learn how to manage your stress: Easier said than done, but read on: it may help !
- Get advice: From an occupational therapist or physiotherapist, or from a back school.
- Lose weight: Especially if there's a pot belly in sight !
- Drink plenty of water every day.
- Take 5/10 minutes a day alone, lie down and think of nothing.

Where does my pain come from ?

- The human spinal column provides support for the head and body and protects the spinal cord.

- The spine needs to be flexible and strong, which is why we have bones called vertebrae, separated by shock absorbers called discs.

- The vertebrae in the neck and lower back regions have greater flexibility which is where problems occur very often.

- In the evolution from monkey to man, the soft discs adapted to support the body weight and the spinal column formed three curves, in the neck, the upper back and lower back.

- We have 24 vertebrae. Muscles and ligaments (or elastic type straps) help to keep the spinal column upright.

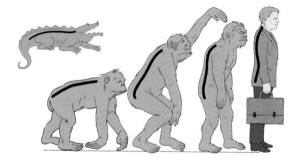

- The discs have a soft interior and a fibrous exterior. After the age of 25, the lubricating fluids in the discs start to dry up and the discs become worn.
- The ageing of discs takes place at different speeds depending on how well or badly we have used them in our lives.
- We can get irritation of nerves around the disc giving local muscle contraction or spasm, called LUMBAGO.
- We can get pressure on a disc which touches a nerve. This can give pain in one or both legs and can be SCIATICA.
- A HERNIATED DISC occurs when fibrous material of the disc wears and the soft material inside the disc is pushed outside.
- ARTHRITIS of the spine is due to ageing of the discs which become thinner, and drier and harder and put more pressure on the articulations of the vertebrae and often on the nerves.

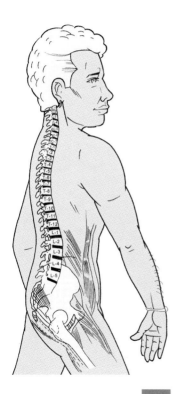

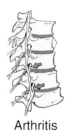

Arthritis

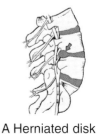

A Herniated disk

WHAT TO DO IF BACK PAIN COMES ON SUDDENLY

 • Sudden pain may be brought on by a bad movement, by overload or by stress. Muscles contract resulting in: stiff neck, upper back pain, lower back pain.

 • As much rest as possible is essential in a position with a firm pillow supporting the neck and back, and a roll or pillow under the knees.
• Use a hot water bottle or heated cushion on the painful area.
• Inform your doctor if the pain persists for longer than 48 hours. He or she may recommend: medication or massage.
• After 24 hours, lying in bed do the following four stretching exercises (see illustrations). If pain increases, do not continue, try again the next day.
• Relax, read or listen to soothing music. It will pass !

EXERCISES TO DO DURING OR AFTER AN ACUTE PHASE OF BACK PAIN, IN BED OR ON AN EXERCISE MAT ON THE FLOOR.

1. On your back with knees bent. Push your back at waist level on to the mattress or mat. Hold and release 3 / 4 times.

2. With knees bent, gently move from left to right, right to left 3 / 4 times.

3. Lying with knees bent. Head on pillow, raise one knee to chest, push right hand/left knee / counter pressure.
Left hand / right knee / counter pressure. 3 / 4 times.

4. Slide upper body from side to side, try to touch your ankle with your hand. 3 / 4 times.

Think of your Body as a Whole

- The ability to relax your mind can also help relax your back and body.
- General stretching or relaxation exercises from head to toe will help to keep the whole body fit.

- Your pain is in one small, specific part of the body, but pain has a habit of shifting to other areas when we try to protect that initial painful area by moving tensely.
- Pain in a knee or ankle joint can often result in back or hip pain.
- Pain in the neck or shoulders may transfer to the upper or lower back or vice versa, especially if we are tense or think negatively.

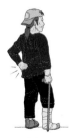

Your Teeth

- Do you grind your teeth ? If the answer is yes then you are probably a tense person, who sleeps and moves in a tense manner and risks back pain problems.
- A tense jaw with clenched teeth sets up tension in the neck, middle of the back and can influence the lower back.

- Check with your dentist to see if your bite is correct. He may suggest using a bite plate especially at night which will stop you grinding and decrease tension.
- Every morning in front of the bathroom mirror make some gentle stretching exercises with your mouth and jaw. Exaggerate pronouncing the vowel sounds AEIOU.

Your Feet

- Bad feet = bad back !!
  How long is it since you looked after your feet ?
  Look at the soles of your shoes. Where are
  they more worn down ? Walking on the outside,
  inside or on your heels can influence your
  posture, creating tension and pain.

- High heeled shoes look fine, but are deadly for
  your back. Choose something with a small heel
  – not a flat shoe without an arch support.

- Remove your shoes, stand on a tennis ball and
  massage your feet. This will show you how to
  feel your pressure points.

- Visit your chiropodist regularly to remove hard
  skin and callouses.

- Wear a pair of sport shoes with a cushion sole
  and arch support, or support sandals around the
  house especially if your floors are hard.

- Put a soft sole insert into your ordinary shoes which will help to absorb shocks on hard pavements. Wear your sports shoes as much as possible when shopping.
- Personalised foot supports may be necessary in case of chronic problems.

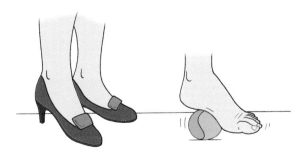

Your Posture

Who are you ? Are your:

• Knees locked back when you stand ? Hips tilted forward, tummy sticking out, lower back arched ? Is your upper back rounded ? Are your shoulders hunched forward or raised upwards tensely ? Are your elbows rigid and your hands clenched especially when you wake up in the morning ? Is your jaw tense ? Do you often have pain in the joints in front of your ears ? Is your head or chin pushed awkwardly forward ?

Or are your:

• Knees slightly bent when you stand ? Your tummy tucked in, your lower back in its natural curve ? Is your upper back straight ? Are your shoulders loose, relaxed and lowered ? Are your elbows bent, your fingers and hands relaxed ? Is your jaw relaxed ? Is your head comfortable with your chin tucked in ?

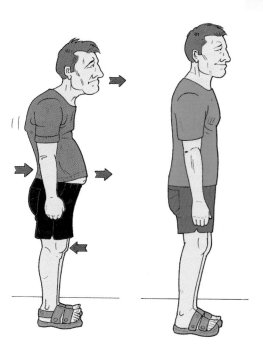

**BEING AWARE OF YOUR POSTURE IS
ALREADY THE FIRST STEP TOWARDS
IMPROVING IT !!**

Stress and Tension

- Alarm rings 6.30, dive out of bed, trip over slippers.
- Early meeting, no time for a shower, certainly no time for exercises.
- Grab coffee.
- Rush out 10 minutes late already.
- Huge traffic jam, swear like mad, bang on horn.
- Park car 15 minutes late.
- Sprint on hard pavements, forget to tie shoelaces, nearly break neck !
- Heavy breathing, sweating, arrive.
- Boss looks furious.
- Open window, so hot, sit in draught.
- Spend whole day on edge of seat, will I get fired ?
- Home 7 pm, no food in fridge, a pile of bills, not enough money to pay them, go to bed, think about boss and money all night.

Next morning, back is killing me, never happened before, wonder why ??

And How to Cope With It

- The alarm rings 6.15, two minutes to lie, reflect on the day and plan, stretch arms, legs, bend knees, flatten lower back at waist on to mattress, breathe in, slowly breathe out.
- Roll out of bed slowly, long hot shower followed by five minutes of stretching exercises on the floor.
- Glass of water or juice with breakfast.
- Leave on time.
- Huge traffic jam, relaxing music tape on the cassette player, have allowed for traffic jam.
- Park car, walk slowly to office, thinking supple, breathing deeply.
- Good morning boss, big smile.
- Sit comfortably at office desk, with good back support, stand up and stretch while on phone.
- Home 6 pm walk slowly to supermarket for shopping, forward plan how to pay bills, relaxed evening meal, to bed with good book for 10 minutes, sleep well.

OR

 • No need for alarm, children, babies all yelling at 6 am, won't eat breakfast, husband has no clean shirts, washing machine breaks down, baby sick, cries all morning, finally get dressed around lunchtime, carry baby on hip and vacuum carpet, change sheets, carry washing downstairs with baby & two children, go to supermarket, lift children in and out of car, lift four bags of groceries, two crates of drinks and carry them up three flights stairs with children. Bathtime for baby who weighs 12 kgs, phone rings, feel like screaming, sudden movement to answer phone, sharp pain, back is blocked !

OR

- No need for alarm, children, babies all yelling at 6am. All into bed with Dad, 15 minutes in bathroom alone for Mum, shower or bath, five minutes of stretching on bathroom floor or other room with door firmly shut, move and dress slowly, deep breathing, drink plenty of water, won't forget to eat. Forward planned the ironing when children were resting, so lots of clean shirts ! Baby is sick so vacuuming can wait. Walk slowly to the supermarket with children, with back pack, buy enough food to fit in back pack, not too heavy, will do a big shop on Saturday with husband. Bathing baby, kneeling on the floor, phone rings but have left answer phone on, will ring back, remember to tighten buttocks and abdominal muscles as I lift baby out of bath, feeling pretty good !

Menopause and Depression

Female and Male:

- Depression, or a feeling of inadequacy, of constant fatigue, of anxiety, of an inability to function normally or cope, of a desire to hide away from the world can happen at any stage in life, but very often occurs with both men and women in their late forties or fifties and is commonly linked with increasing aches and pains, particularly back pain.

- Menopause or the change of life is physically linked with a change in our hormonal structure in both males and females, but outside factors also may play a significant role at this time of life.

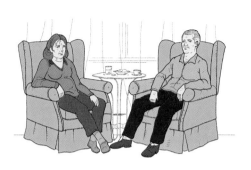

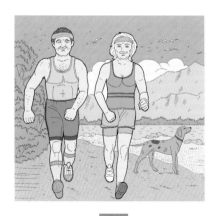

Males

- So you've hit 50, your hair is thinning, the belt that once fastened around the waist has shifted down a few cms below the pot belly. They don't want you anymore at work, you are too old or not fit enough and the opposite sex don't look at you like they used to ! You are worried and tense, its another 15 years till retirement, you have so many financial burdens, or you cannot cope with the physical demands of your work. So you have another glass of wine or a whisky while you think about it. Suddenly your back feels painful in the mornings, something has to be done! You inscribe at the gym, throw yourself madly into a programme of body building made for 30 year olds, or you go on a 10km run with no preparations, you block your back, end up in bed for two weeks and you feel depressed !

- So you've hit 50, and you are going to pace yourself in life. If you've had no time for sport or exercise before, now is the time to start but slowly ! Walk briskly for one hour twice a week on soft ground with a good pair of sports shoes, swing your arms. Empty your mind, think of nothing, look around you at nature – it costs nothing. Seek professional advice, learn how to stretch and relax your muscles before any sporting activity. Shower immediately after exertion that makes you sweat. Give yourself time and space to relax, watch your diet and alcohol intake. Have regular medical check ups.

Accept your age: you'll live longer if you do !

Females

- Your children have left home, all of a sudden you hear clocks ticking, its so quiet, you feel your major role in life is over. Overnight your entire wardrobe no longer fits, you hate looking in the mirror. All the young mothers pushing prams look like school children. Your back is stiff in the mornings, hurts when you do the housework, you can't find a comfortable seat anymore. You feel miserable.

- You may have more time on your hands, so use it.
- For 15 minutes each day, lie on your bed or sofa with a firm support under neck and upper back, lower back flat, use a hot water bottle or heated cushion if your back is painful. Your knees should be bent with a roll or cushion support. Listen to music, read or sleep.
- Walk briskly at least 1/2 hour per day on soft ground, use sports shoes with plantar support and swing your arms. Empty your head, think of nothing.
- Get a dog if you feel lonely, but keep him or her on a short leash and close to you, it is better for your back.
- Intellectual and physical stimulation from hobbies, clubs or sports are excellent ways of maintaining a healthy mind, but remember to change your position frequently if sitting or standing to help maintain a healthy back.

Diet

- Too many sweet and fatty foods, just another glass of wine or beer, not enough plain water, irregular meal times may all lead to digestive problems, weight problems, back problems and other health risks.

- If you feel thirsty, you have already left it too late !

- Drink at least one litre of water per day in frequent small quantities, before you feel thirsty.

- Three balanced meals a day will help you to maintain a healthy body.

Smoking

- **IT'S SIMPLE, DON'T !**
  Not only do you risk drying up all the lubricating fluids in the discs between your vertebrae, but you risk killing yourself and everyone else around you.

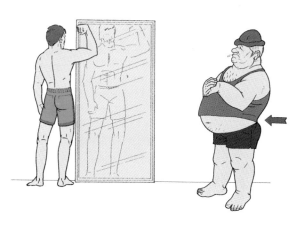

The Pelvic Tilt

Certain groups of muscles in our back may become shorter and tighter than others, often this is due to lack of exercise or stretching and bad postural habits. This may result in you having a pelvis pushed upwards and backwards causing a "flat back", or if your pelvis is pushed forward and downwards you will have a "sway back".

In order to maintain a healthy back when performing our activities of daily living, we need to keep a flexible pelvic girdle. It is one of those parts of the body we tend to forget about (until our backs hurt !), but keeping the pelvis supple should be part of a daily exercise routine.

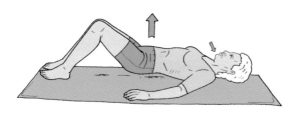

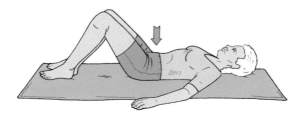

Understanding the Feeling of a Flexible, Supple Pelvic Girdle (Pelvic Tilt)

Lie on your back on the floor, knees bent, make a double chin. Lift your hips off the ground to horizontal, count to six. Slowly push your hips down until your back touches the floor. Tighten your abdominal muscles and push your back at waist or belt level (not your buttocks) on to the ground. Hold to the count of six and release.

Or

Stand against a wall, shoulders against the wall, knees bent, feet 30 cm from the wall. Make a double chin, and flatten your whole back against the wall, count to six and release.
• To make sure you have done this properly, ask someone to try to slide their hand between your back and the wall at waist height, if they can't you have done the exercise correctly.
• Making a double chin with shoulders against the wall will also make sure that your head and neck are in a correct position.

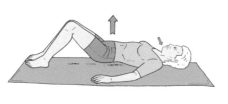

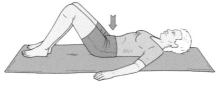

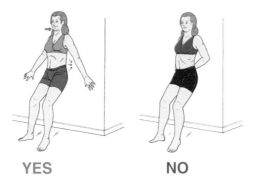

YES **NO**

At Home

General Rules

- Think about your back, am I comfortable ?
  Listen to your back, I am in pain, why ?
  Think **supple**, think **straight**, think **close**, work
  your legs to protect your back.

- Don't ignore a niggling back pain, it will get
  worse if you do nothing about it. Don't do too
  much in a day, a sudden onset of back pain for
  no reason is your body telling your mind to slow
  down ! Don't sit or stand for long periods
  without changing position.
  Avoid extreme movements.

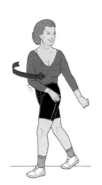

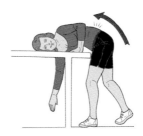

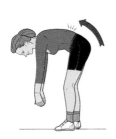

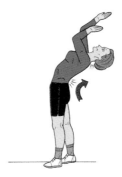

Beds and Bedrooms

- We spend about 1/3 of our lives in bed.
- We may turn or move up to 250 times per night, which is why the average life span of a mattress is 8 years.

- Choose a bed base which is flexible, moving when you move. Choose a mattress which moulds to your body – not too hard, nor too soft. If you sleep with a partner, make sure you have two mattresses on one bed base each adapted to your own weight.
- Sleep with a therapeutic pillow which fills the curve of your neck.

- Do not choose a bed with a rigid base or rigid wooden slats.
- Do not choose a mattress that is too hard or too soft
- Your bed should not be too low. A bed base 30 cms from the ground is a reasonable height.
- Don't sleep in a draught. Backs should be kept warm at night. Sleeping with no pillow or one or two soft feather pillows give no support to the neck. Avoid them !

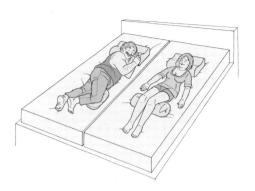

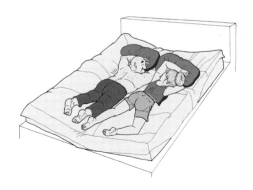

In Bed

- To get into bed: sit on the edge of the bed, help with your hands if your bed is low, lean on **both** arms lifting legs on to the bed (one movement), lie down on your side, knees bent. To turn on to your back, imagine your knees are glued together. Roll over in one movement, shoulders and hips at the same time. Reverse procedure to **get out** of bed.

- Getting into bed violently, lying down directly from sitting position, leaving one leg behind on the floor are all excellent ways to ruin your back !

THINK SUPPLE !

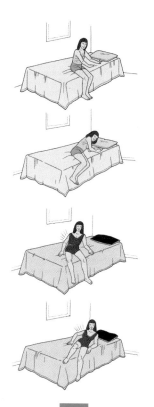

Sleeping Positions

- On your back, head supported with a good pillow, knees bent with a roll support. Check that your back at waist height is resting on mattress.
- On your side, good pillow, upper leg forward of lower leg which enables the hips to be relaxed. Use a pillow to support upper leg if necessary.

- Avoid sleeping without a pillow, or with too many soft pillows.
- Avoid sleeping on your back with legs straight, this arches the lower back and gives no lumbar support.
- Avoid sleeping on your stomach. This position exaggerates the lumbar curve, tires the neck and shoulders and impedes breathing. If you have to sleep like this, put a soft cushion under your stomach.

Material
Orthopaedic pillow
Knee Roll
Supple Mattress / Bed Base

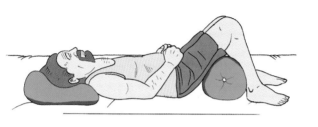

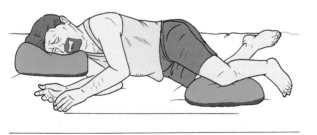

Your Sex Life

- There are numerous ways to express love and have pleasure without killing your back. There is not a position **not recommended**.
Be inventive and look for comfort and enjoyment

- Lying on your side, or sitting and lying may be preferable at certain times.

- Avoid any extreme position, particularly hyper extension of your lower back.

THINK SUPPLE !

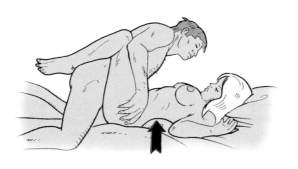

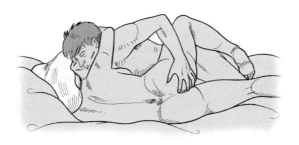

The Bathroom

The first two or three hours of the day after getting up are the most risky for your back, so pay attention, particularly when you go into the bathroom.

- What do you normally do ? Look in mirror, yawn, bend over the basin with round back and knees locked, and wash your face. Come up abruptly to grab toothpaste or razor and repeat movement; knees locked, round back etc. etc. HIGH RISK !

- What you should do ! Look in mirror, yawn, lean on one hand on basin, bend knees, put one foot on the small stool (opposite foot to leaning hand) under the basin. Bend over, come up and repeat several times with no risk to your lower back. Change leaning hand and foot regularly.

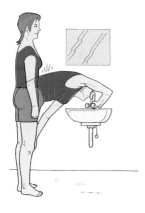
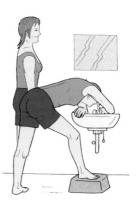

- The shower with a non slip mat is a less risky place for your back than the bath. Try to wash your hair in the shower. If you use a bath, use hand rails, keep knees bent, tighten tummy and buttocks when you lower in and come out of the bath.

- What do your normally do ? Need to wash your hair in a hurry. Grab the shower attachment in the bath, knees are locked, lean over rounding back, wash hair, twisting at the same time to find the shampoo and the towel. Wonder why it hurts when try to stand up. HIGH RISK !

- What you should do ! Small people should lean with one hand on opposite side of the bath, rest opposite knee against the bath, then round back to wash hair. Towel and shampoo within reach. Tall people should kneel on floor on a towel, lean against bath and wash hair. Hands on edge of bath to push up to standing position.

I need:
A small stool 10-15 cms high
Non slip mats
Hand rails on bath
Older People
A bath board or/and bench to slide into the bath or
a stool in the shower. Hand rails near toilet and
bath.

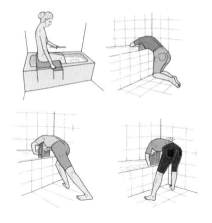

Shoes, Socks, Tights and Toenails

 • Usual scenario ! Slept through the alarm, dive out of bed, quick shower, back stiff !! Tights/socks in the bottom of the lowest cupboard, search for shoes at the back of wardrobe, knees locked back, round back. Move tensely and quickly. Back even stiffer. Cannot even reach my knees let alone bend down to put on socks/tights or shoes. Help !

 • Try this for a change ! Slept through the alarm, roll out of bed, think supple ! Quick shower, two or three stretching exercises. Kneel on floor to find tights/socks. Move close to wardrobe kneeling, find shoes. Thinking about tilting my pelvis, tightening abdominals and buttocks, straight back. Put on socks/tights/shoes using most comfortable method:
• Stand, arm against wall or stand back against wall.
• Lying on bed on back or side.
• Sitting on chair, crossed leg. Sitting on chair using a stocking aid, or long handled aid.
• Sitting on stairs, or standing at bottom of stairs, one foot up two steps. Standing one foot on a stool.

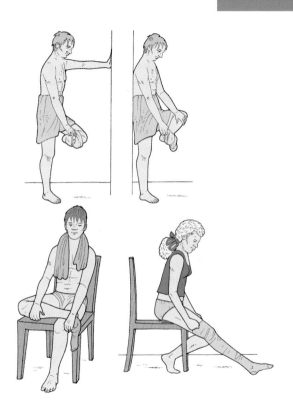

Dress

- It's the image that counts !
  Squeeze into pencil line tight skirt, belt slightly uncomfortable so need to breathe in all day. Jacket is really tight round shoulders – but goes well with the skirt. Finishing touches are the narrow high heeled shoes. Perfect ! Ignore the tension in the neck or lower back.

- Simplify life, you can still be smart but comfortable. Choose textiles and cuts of clothes which permit free movement to bend, to kneel, to stretch, to lift.
- Make sure your neck and lower back are well protected against cold or draughts.
- What you put on your feet can be partly responsible for encouraging good or bad posture, no pain or pain in neck/shoulders and lower back.
- Choose shoes with a heel of between two and four cms / no more / no less. Avoid laces. Use cushion sole inserts to absorb shocks or choose shoes with built in plantar supports.

Helpful Aids for Dressing

Long handled shoe horn
Long handled pincher or stocking aid
Stool 10-15 cms high
Shoe or boot remover

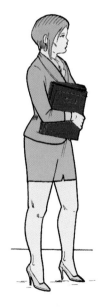
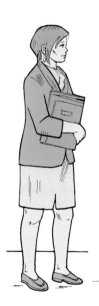

Useful Positions to Adopt When Doing Housework or Performing Heavy Activities

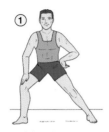

(1)

tighten buttocks

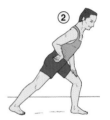

(2)

tighten buttocks or
one hand leaning on wall

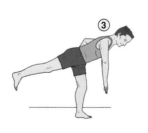

(3)

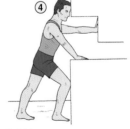

(4)

Back remains straight

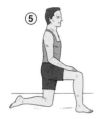
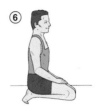

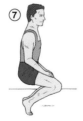

Back remains straight

In the Kitchen

A few facts:

- We are growing taller as generations go on. Unfortunately our work surfaces are generally too low. Stand upright, bend your elbow at a right angle. Your kitchen top should be between 5-10 cms lower than your elbow bent at 90°.
- If your work top is too low, buy some thick wooden chopping boards. This will help raise the level while you are preparing food.
- Avoid constantly bending to reach your favourite cup or casserole in the back of the most inaccessible cupboard.
- Avoid stretching to the top shelf of the cupboard for the salt or sugar that you use several times a day.
- Organise your favourite cups and casseroles, and products that you use often to be somewhere easy at hand, not too low not too high.
- For all low cupboards or ovens, bend at knees, straight back, tighten your buttocks and tummy muscles, kneel on all fours, or one knee on the ground, **keep close**. ⚠ *pos. 5/6/7 page 71.*
- For all high cupboards, tighten tummy muscles. Use a step stool. ⚠

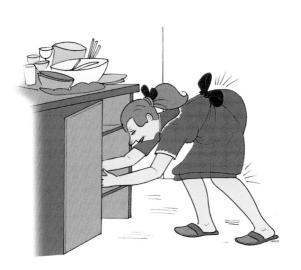

At the Sink

- Its 11pm, the day has been hard and you are exhausted. Still a pile of dishes to wash. You are tense and you hurry. Your knees are locked back, lower back is arched. The sink is too low, you bend your back, rush through the dishes and can hardly straighten up when they are finished !

- Its 11pm, the day has been hard and you are exhausted ! You have two washing up bowls in your sink. One is upturned, the bigger one sits on the other so you have raised the level of your sink. You open the cupboard door, put one foot at the bottom shelf, or put one foot on the small stool in front of you and you lean against the sink. You wash up, from time to time resting your forehead on the kitchen cupboard above you, changing as well the foot resting on the stool or shelf. You think straight, close and supple.

Try positions 1 or 4 (page 70) with stool. For long periods of standing – break off and do the pelvic tilt exercise against a wall. Page 50-51.

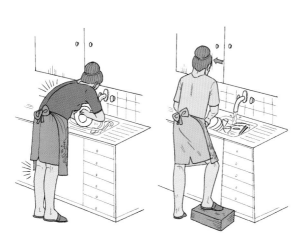

The Oven or Dishwasher

- The oven door opens forwards. You bend over, legs straight, pick up a heavy casserole, stand up abruptly, twist without moving your feet and put it on the counter almost behind you.
  HIGH RISK !

- The oven door opens forwards. You kneel on one knee to the side of the oven. You remove the heavy casserole, place it on the work surface immediately in front of you, without moving your position. You stand up and face the counter.
  LOW RISK !

Try position 5 (page 71)

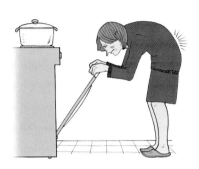

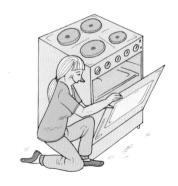

Preparing Food

- Dinner to prepare for eight, vegetables to peel and chop, meat to slice, soup to simmer, salad to wash, cakes to mix. At least an hour's work and your back already hurts. HIGH RISK !

- Lean !
  - Against the cupboard, on work surface, one foot on a small stool or on a lower shelf.
  - Lean with one hand on the work top whilst you stir the soup.
  - Rest your head against the cupboard in front of you.

- Sit on a high stool, preferably one which will tilt forward, keep close to the work surface.

- Every few minutes, stop what you are doing, walk round the room, STRETCH / exercise against the wall ◭ *(page 50-51).*

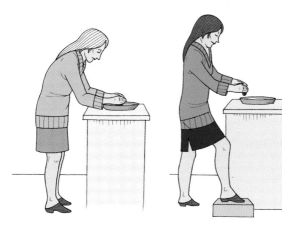

Shopping

- You jump in the car, drive for five minutes to the supermarket. Grab a caddy, has a stiff wheel but if you push and twist a bit it works alright. Your shoulder bag contains two purses, cheque book, mobile phone, calculator, pens, make up, passports, diary etc. You put it on the right shoulder, it always drops off the left and off you go ! Bending, stretching, pushing, pulling, lifting and twisting – the usual gestures in the super market. You only have one shopping bag, so you pack it all in tight, lift from the cash desk to the caddy, from the caddy to the car, from the car to the front door step, front door to the kitchen floor, and then you unpack, bending, twisting, stretching and lifting ! OUCH !!

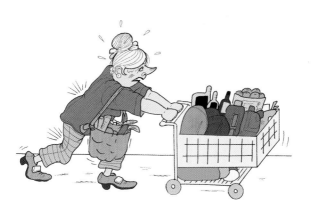

• You walk for 10 minutes to the supermarket because you don't need too much shopping today. You choose a caddy that runs smoothly ! Your bag with two shoulder straps contains all the usual items but is equally weighted on both shoulders, or you change shoulders regularly if you have a shoulder bag. You remember when you are pulling, pushing, bending and lifting to think of your pelvic tilt exercise. You tighten your tummy and buttock muscles and use *pos 2/3/7 page 70-71*. You've brought two shopping bags so you pack equal weights. Walking home you remember to tuck in your elbows to your waist, this takes the strain off shoulders and the neck, you carry with your forearms.

• Shopping goes on the work top and you unpack from there.

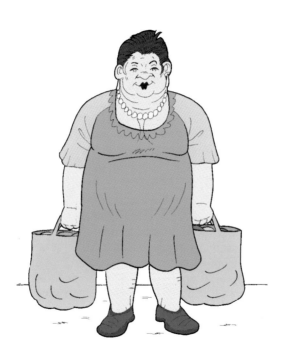

Housework

THINK STRAIGHT, THINK CLOSE, THINK SUPPLE !

Making Beds

- You hate making beds, so want to do it quickly. Your bed is in a corner, so with great effort you stretch violently, lift the corner of the heavy mattress, attempt to tuck the sheet in, and then you bend, tuck in, stand up, bend, tuck in, stand up etc. at great speed. Your legs are rigid, knees locked back, you collapse on the bed with back pain !

- You hate making beds, and know it's a high risk factor for your back. You choose fitted sheets and duvet covers. You move round the bed, with one knee on the ground *(position 5)*, on all fours *(ref. Page 70-71, position 6)*, or with one knee leaning against the mattress *(position 1)*. You kneel on the bed and get close to the difficult corner. You don't lift the mattress or you get help to do so. ⚠️You lean with one hand on the bed or the wall where possible *(positions 2)*.

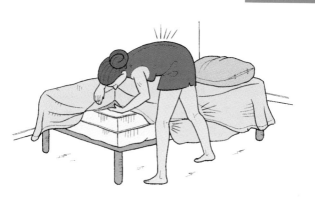

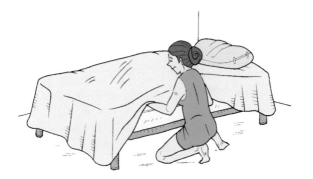

Sweeping, Vacuuming, Cleaning the Bath

- Your mother-in-law will be here in half an hour, the flat looks like a bomb has hit it. You pull out the vacuum cleaner in great haste, race around the flat, bend under the table, bend under the sofa, bend under the beds, twisting violently to avoid furniture. Phew ! Now for the bathroom ! Lean over the bath, rubbing furiously the tide marks. You are crippled when mother in law arrives and have to go to bed early !

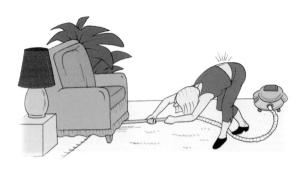

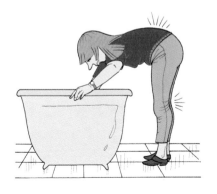

- Your mother-in-law will be here in half an hour, the flat looks like a bomb hit it ! You remove the vacuum cleaner remembering to keep your tummy and buttock muscles tight, knees slightly bent, protecting your back, when you pull it from the cupboard.
- You move around the room *(pos 2) page 70-71* keeping the cylinder and the tube close to you, use *(pos 5)* to move under furniture.
- To sweep or wash the floor use the same positions, putting your pail of water on a low stool to avoid bending.
- Using a dustpan and brush *(pos 5 or 6)* or use one with long handles.
- Now for the bath ! Take *pos 6 or pos 2* lean against the bath, with one hand on the opposite side, changing knee and hand as you clean. Mother in law arrives and you are on top form !

THINK CLOSE, THINK STRAIGHT, THINK SUPPLE

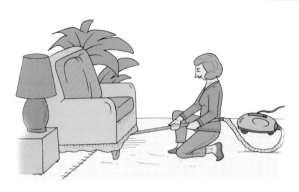

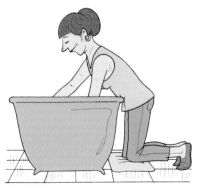

The Washing Machine and Ironing

- You pile 10 days worth of washing into the basket, round back, straight legs. You have three flights of stairs down to the machine, basket in front of you or on one hip, lower back arched. Everything on to the floor, lean over, pick up, lean over, pick up and twist a few times !

- You split the load, carry the basket in front of you, tightening tummy and buttock muscles. Three flights of stairs twice but that's good exercise ! Basket on to a work top – load the machine standing *pos 1 or 2* or putting basket on the floor, *pos 5 page 70-71.*

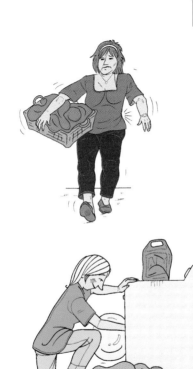

• You've let the ironing build up, have allocated two hours to finish it. Your board is too low and does not adjust. You go hard at it, knees locked back, lower back arched, neck bent ! After two hours you can hardly move !

 • You've let the ironing build up, but you'll do one hour today, one hour tomorrow. Your board adjusts. Check your arm at right angle – board is 5-10 cms below your bent arm. You have a small stool to put your foot on. You change feet every five minutes or you have a higher stool and rest your knee on it, changing every five minutes. You move round the room frequently, putting away the ironing. After one hour you are fine !

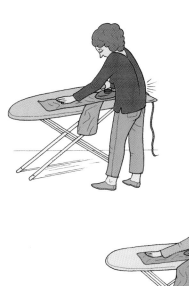
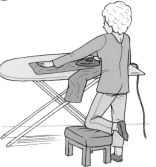

Eating and at the Table

- You've had a hard day, all you want to do is relax in front of the TV. You perch on the end of the sofa, tray on the low coffee table, you lean forward, your tummy is squashed, back rounded, you eat your meal and end up with a bad back and indigestion. *or*
- You have inherited some old wooden high backed chairs from Grandma and your dining table doesn't match so it is too high or too low. The chair is rigid, uncomfortable, gives no support and after an hour at table your back is totally stiff !

- For the sake of good digestion, you eat at a proper table. Check correct table height, sit with arms by your side, the height of your table should correspond with the bend in your arm at elbow level. *or*
- You still have the inherited old wooden chairs, but you have cushions on the seats, and have purchased firm back support cushions which give your back something to lean against, and you rest your feet on the wooden support under the table.

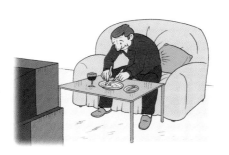

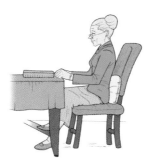

Armchairs and Relaxing

- You sink into the soft old armchair, and you stretch out your feet on the coffee table. Your legs are straight, there's a huge gap at lower back level, the chair pushes your upper back and neck forward, after 15 minutes everything hurts !

or

- You are going to relax in front of the TV. You lie on your stomach, on the floor, back and neck arched – as a child there's no problem to get up, a teenager may have a stiff neck, an adult will probably need a pick up fork lift to prise you off the floor !

- You sink into the soft old armchair, where you have ready waiting your firm back support cushion which fills in the gap ! You put a cushion or roll under your knees before you put your feet on the coffee table, or you have a leg rest support which keeps knees bent and releases tension in the lower back.

For an adult, if you are going to relax in front of the TV, lie on the sofa, back and neck supported, roll under your knees. The TV is in front of you, so you don't twist your head. For a child, lie on your stomach on a large bean bag or an orthopaedic ball and keep moving !

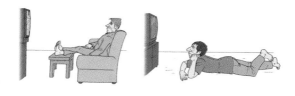

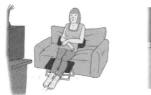
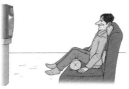

Pregnancy

- The weight of the unborn baby increases the curve in your lower back pulling your pelvis down and forward and may result in backache and sciatica.

- Whether sitting, standing or lying, try to maintain a flexible pelvic girdle and practice frequently the exercises on *page 166-169*. Keep tummy and buttock muscles tight when you exert an effort, and use your legs *(all positions on page 70-71)* in order to protect your back.

- Take the time to rest during the day.

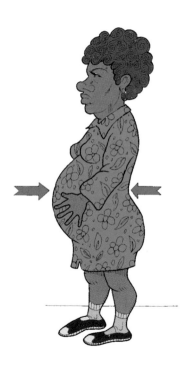

Babies and Children

- You are tired out, the baby is crying again. You struggle out of bed, you lean over the cot rail, bend back, straight legs and lift the baby who suddenly feels very heavy. Your nursing chair is an old one with not much back or elbow support. Baby is fed, time for a bath. Your bath is a deep, old fashioned variety. You lean, you bend, you wash, you lift and twist to reach a towel. You lie baby on your bed and repeat. You lean, you bend, you twist and you lift. Baby is clean and smiling, Mum is groaning in pain. You pop baby on your right hip and carry him round most of the day because he's teething and won't be put down. To get a bit of rest you bend to put him on the floor, two minutes later you are bending to pick him up again !

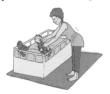
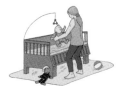

Remember to
THINK STRAIGHT, SUPPLE AND CLOSE

You are tired out, the baby is crying again. You roll out of bed. Your cot has an adaptable rail which you lower. You get as close to him as you can, you lift him using *pos 1 or 2 page 70-71*. Your nursing chair has a good high back, lumbar support and cushions to support your elbows. Baby is fed, time for a bath. You have a baby bath on a frame or placed on a high surface. You fill the bath with a hose or a pail and bathe him standing up, keeping close, or you kneel *(pos 5/6)* whilst he's in the bath. You have a stool close by to sit on and dry him. Alternatively, you have a bath with him, you have a non-slip mat in the bath, you keep him on your knees and use a hand rail to help stand up. You lie baby on a changing table, ideal height 90 cm. Keeping your baby close and taking *pos 1 or 2*, you can change and dress him without hurting your back.

Carry your child in front of you in the first weeks using the special, adapted carry bags or on your back when he's older. Hold him on your hip, but keep your upper body straight, and change hips. To lift him from the ground take *pos 5 or 7 page 71* – tighten tummy and buttock muscles △ as you lift. Make sure your feet are well apart. Lift him on to your knee and hug him close as you stand up. As your baby starts to walk and needs to hold your hands, use a harness with a strap on those days when your back is painful.

YOUR CHILD'S BACK IS AS IMPORTANT AS YOURS. TRY TO TEACH HIM WHAT YOU ARE LEARNING, THEN HE WON'T NEED THIS BOOK WHEN HE'S AN ADULT ! YOU CAN ALSO REMEMBER HOW TO MAKE MOVEMENTS CORRECTLY BY OBSERVING YOUR TODDLER.

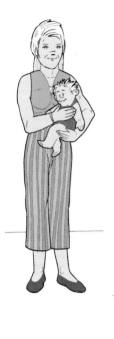
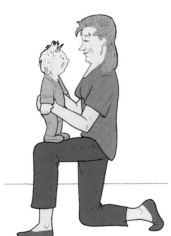

A FEW FACTS:

- Did you know that in the Western world four out of five people every day see their doctor or therapist as a result of a bad back and consequently, that on average in European countries 50-100,000 people are off work every day because of back pain !

- Did you know that it is one and a half times more stressful for your back to sit, than to stand, walk or lie down !

- Did you know that when you sit and look at a document, the moment your eyes look more than 30% below horizontal your neck and shoulder muscles work eight times harder than if your eye level remained horizontal !

- Did you know that in Third World countries people have fewer instances of back pain, because the average person is more active, moves constantly, walks a lot and squats to perform certain tasks.
- In Western society, our work often demands static, repetitive movements.
- We have not learned to adapt either our work place or our working methods.
- We are under increasing pressure to perform, thus producing increased stress levels.

A Word About Eyesight

It is important to check your eyesight particularly if you read or study, if you work with computers or if your work involves precision. Using bifocal lenses can increase neck fatigue. Progressive lenses teach you to raise and lower your eyes rather than your head when reading but are not always recommended for work at the computer.

Sitting

We can adopt three types of positions when sitting.

 A good working, studying position needs:

- Table at correct height, check when sitting, arm by your side, table top should be at the same height as the bend in your arm at the elbow. Adjust your chair, or the height of your table.
- An adjustable seat on your chair, either you tilt forward, use a knee seat, a wedge cushion or your legs are bent under the seat and you lean forward.
- You can also place a cushion between your tummy and the table – this keeps your back straight.
- You also need for the sake of your neck and shoulders to work on an inclined surface, around 12-15° is about right.

A listening position needs:

- A chair which gives good lumbar support as well as good upper back support.
- The use of an adjustable foot rest helps your lower back to be firmly supported against the chair back.
- An adjustable tilting chair is ideal.

A resting position needs:

- A chair with neck and upper back support, lower back support and leg and knee support.

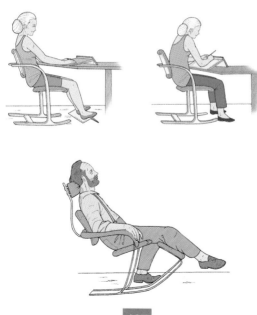

Sitting at a Computer

A typical scene:

* Your desk is rather small, so your computer screen is at an angle and has no filter, your keyboard is on a lower shelf where there is no room to rest your arms and wrists, so there's not much room to get your legs under the desk and you cross them. Your boss hasn't changed the office chairs for years, so yours is soft, has bumps in all the wrong places and doesn't adjust. Your chair is on wheels, so you spend your time moving round the office sitting instead of standing up and changing position. You have a pile of documents to look at – all of them flat on the desk and you'll be at it for at least six hours. You have a large fluorescent strip light on the ceiling and window in front of you.

After six to eight hours at your desk:
* Your lower back is painful,
* Your neck and shoulders are stiff, you have pain between your shoulder blades,
* Your wrists and elbows hurt,
* You have a splitting headache and you are TENSE !

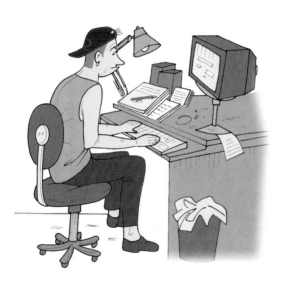

Ideal conditions:

- Desk gives enough space to have screen with a filter directly in front of you.
- Your head is comfortable when looking at the screen and is not tilted up or down, your chin is not pushed forward.
- Keyboard is on a table at the right height for you *(check page 106)*.
- There is space on the table to rest your forearms.
- Wrist support pad for the mouse.
- Documents on a support stand at eye level.
- Sit on an adjustable firm chair, with good upper/lower back support. Seat adjusts forwards/backwards (if not use wedges or back support cushions).
- Adjustable foot rest support.
- Good lighting but not too strong over screen, not too close to windows causing reflections on screen.
- If you need glasses, your optician can recommend the correct lenses for work at a computer screen.

• You don't work for long periods without standing up, walking round making your phone calls and stretching *(exercises on page 166-167 for sitting)*. After six to eight hours at your desk, you are in perfect shape to take a healthy walk !

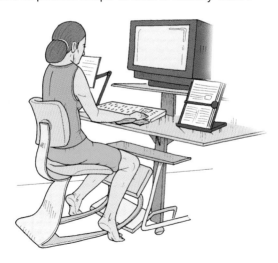

Chairs, Seats and Cushions

THE MORE YOUR BODY CAN MOVE WITH YOUR CHAIR THE BETTER IT IS.

Ideal chairs or seats for working with should have some of these factors:

- Be stable and adjustable in height,
- A seat which can tilt forward and back,
- A moving back rest adjustable in height and depth.

Other alternatives are:

- Knee chairs which are adjustable in height are good for tilting the pelvis forward and taking pressure off lumbar vertebrae but are not recommended for people with knee or circulatory problems.
- Saddle stools adjustable in height and those that tilt forward are ideal for a semi-sitting / standing position.
- Wedge cushions or firm back supports with adjustments. Firm forms for chairs can all be experimented with to find personal comfort.

- Avoid static chairs and static positions.
  KEEP MOVING !

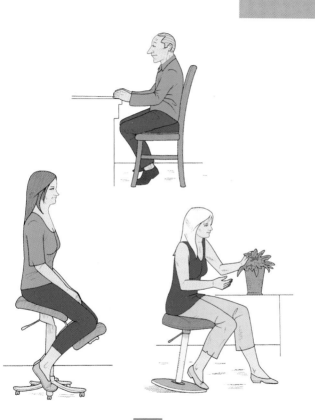

Young People's Backs, Schools and Studying

It is interesting to observe when a young child who automatically moves in a supple way suddenly adopts postures that are potential risks for his back. It is most certainly related to the day he starts school, when he is obliged to sit at a desk for several hours a day and starts suffering from the stresses of life !

- Most school furniture adapts insufficiently to growing children's needs. Chairs are rigid, regulation height for everyone. Tables are flat, children are forced to bend over their desks, backs and heads bent forward.
- This pattern repeats itself very often in Universities and Colleges where furniture may have been purchased economically.

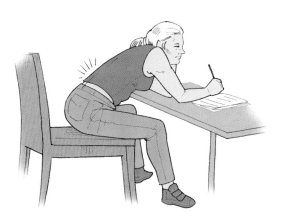

- Luckily, most schools offer regular medical check ups where back problems such as scoliosis, a lateral curve of the spine can be recognised early and treated.

- The same rules that apply to sitting at computers should be applied in schools, and should include inclining tops of desks, adjustable chairs and tables.

- By at least supplying a good study area at home for your child, you are assisting in reducing the percentage of potential back sufferers in adult life.

Materials Needed for Young People Studying

1. Adjustable tilting chair - or orthopaedic ball to sit on.
2. Table or desk adjustable height.
3. Inclined surface for reading or writing.

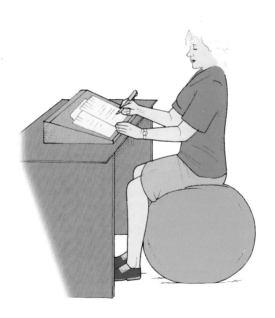

Standing at Work

- You work at the local department store that's sadly in need of renovation. The area where you work is narrow and there are two or three people in the same place. The cash register is in a corner, the counters are low. You stand relatively still for most of the day, you twist to use the cash register, you bend to search for the bags on a low shelf knocking into your colleagues, and you are obliged to wear "smart shoes" for the sake of the shop's image. Your lower back by the end of the day is stiff and sore.

or

- You work at a factory or an assembly line. The work is dirty, noisy and dusty. You repeat the same movements all day long, your head is bent, your work moves from left to right, you are tall and the assembly line or work top is too low. At the end of the day your neck is stiff and you have pain in the upper back and shoulders.

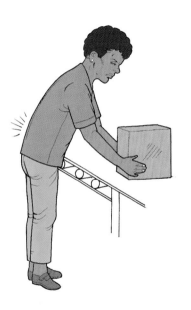

Standing at Work

- The general rule for working and standing is that the table top should be 5 to 10 cms below your elbow bent at a right angle. The heavier the work the lower the height should be, the lighter and more precise the work, the higher the height should be.
- Always look for something to put a foot on, a bar, a box, a stool, a book of about 10-15 cms and change feet regularly.
- Lean against the work top, adopt *pos 1 or 2, page 70*
- Use an adjustable tilting stool if you can.
- Sit or change your position when you take a break.
- Do one or two of the stretching exercises for standing on *page 168-169* and do the ⚠ against a wall.
- Wear comfortable shoes, preferably with a plantar support that helps to soften hard floors.

- If you are a nurse or a waiter or in one of the professions where you stand, but move a lot and lift a lot - you are in fact luckier than most. The static positions are most harmful to your back. But be aware that comfortable shoes can help, that stopping for a minute to make the pelvic tilt against a wall and adopting *position 2/3, page 70* will help you take the strain.

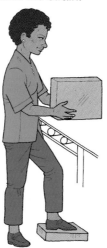

Standing at Parties

- It's the office party. There are 150 people in a large room. You've made an effort - so out the high heels have come. Your shoulder bag is too heavy and you have a drink in the other hand. You have been engaged in conversation with the most boring person for at least 1/2 an hour and you don't think your back will stand another minute ! Your knees are locked and you are tense. You shuffle in a military stance. Stand on one leg, stick out a hip and arch your lower back - you want to go home !

- Be reasonable, choose a pair of shoes with a slightly lower heel. Try to keep to the edges of the room where you can lean on a table, lean on a wall, put your heel against the wall. Practice the pelvic tilt, tightening your buttocks and tummy muscles without leaning against the wall - no one will notice ! Think supple - even though you are bored ! Keep moving, talking to other people ! Had a good evening ?!

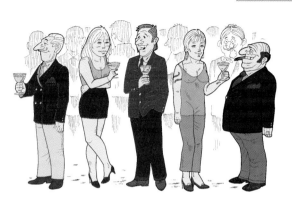

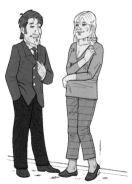

LIFTING AND MOVING

A few facts:

- Most back injuries are as a result of lifting badly, or lifting quickly without thinking about your back.

- Take a weight of 25 kgs, when you push it on a trolley, there is no weight supported by your back. Lifting 25 kgs correctly means that your back has to support a weight of 75 kgs. If you lift badly 25kgs, your back has to support a weight of 375 kgs !! Bear these facts in mind before you lift and practice with an empty box before attempting to lift something heavy.

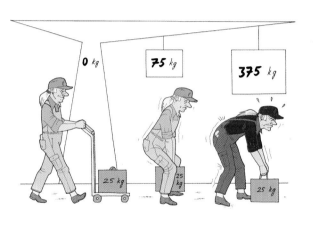

Lifting Light Objects

- Count or write down how many times you bend over in the day to pick up a pen, a piece of paper or other light objects. You will be horrified ! How many times did you bend without putting pressure on your lower back ?

- To save your back, keep it straight, use your legs, lean on a hand, use *positions 2 or 3 (page 70)* for small light objects.

- Try to keep things that you use frequently at table height.

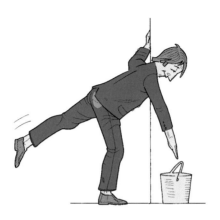

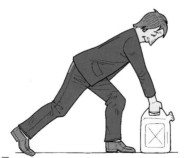

Pre-planned Lifting of Medium/Heavy Objects

- Think before you act. Look for obstacles that may be in your way. Choose the flattest surface possible. Be comfortable in your clothes that have no loose flaps, wear gloves if necessary. Make sure you have stable non slip shoes. Can I pick up this load at about 60-90 cms off the floor and put it down at the same height ?
Think how much this load weighs - can I split it ?
Do I need help ? Can I re-organise my environment so that I don't always need to be lifting these loads ?

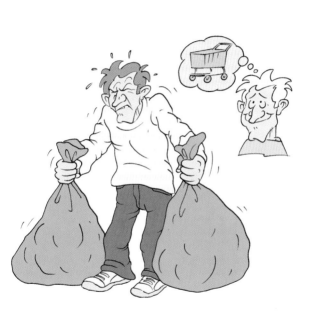

Lifting Properly Medium / Heavy Objects

KEEP STRAIGHT; KEEP CLOSE

- Practice these moves using an empty box, before you attempt a heavy load.
- Spread feet well apart.
- Approach the object to be close to your centre of gravity.
- Face the way you want to move.
- Keep close to a wall that you can use to lean on if necessary.
- Put one knee on the floor keeping back straight.
- Tighten buttocks, tighten abdominal muscles.
- Using the pelvic tilt ◮ lift the object on to your raised knee, "hug" your load.
- Using the pelvic tilt ◮ stand up or slide up the wall letting your leg muscles work.
- Grasp your load firmly with both hands, move slowly forward, don't twist.
- Try to put your load down at waist height.
- Use mechanical help and the help of others for larger, more difficult objects.

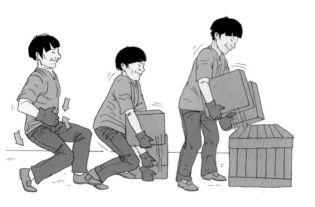

Moving House - Pushing, Pulling and Lifting

- There are very few activities worse for your mind, body and back than moving house ! You are usually highly stressed, with too much to do in too little time, and very often financially ruined ! You are buying or renting a new house, you need a new bed, a new washing machine etc etc. So how do you save money - by doing the move yourself ! You rent a van, bribe a couple of friends to help and you are so pleased to have saved some cash ! For three or four days, you sweat, you push, you pull, you heave, you lift, you bend and twist, twist and bend and two days later instead of enjoying the new home, you are stuck in bed unable to move !

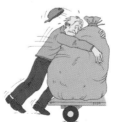

- Try where possible to plan this move several weeks or even months in advance. Pace yourself by doing a little packing each day. Be realistic about how much you put in a box - you should be able to lift it comfortably. Save on the washing machine, not the move.
  Get professional help, certainly for large items.

PUSH, DON'T PULL, BUT KEEP CLOSE.

Flatten your back against the object and push with your legs or push with your hands and legs *(pos 1 and 2, page 70)*, keeping close. Lifting heavy bags - try to have an equal weight on both sides. Tuck in your elbows at waist/hip height to prevent shoulder and neck strain. This way you'll be able to appreciate your new home without having to spend a week in the bedroom !

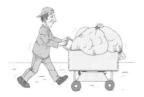

Lifting Children and Adults

 • Watch your toddler lifting something:- they stand in front and over the object keeping close. They bend at the knees, putting their hands under the object. They hug the object using their legs to lift themselves up. As they let go of the object they will often let it slide down their bodies and legs. Copy this "natural method" when lifting your children and you will be protecting your back.

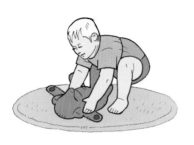

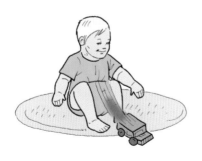

- You may need to help ageing parents or be employed in one of the caring professions. If you don't take care of your back and body, your family, your parents and your work will suffer. Wherever possible, be sure there are two people to lift and transfer.

- Sitting transfers: Ask your relative or patient to assist you as much as possible by moving to the front of the seat. Stand in front of your patient, close and slightly to the side, *pos 1, page 70.* Put one foot in front of their feet, your leg against their knees, keeping your knees flexed, back straight, hold onto the patient's belt or waistband firmly. The patient leans slightly forward and pushes themselves up as you lift.

- In and Out of Beds: The relative or patient should sit on the edge of the bed, shuffling themselves back so they are firmly on the bed. Bend your knees, lean with your knees and thighs against the bed. *Pos 1 page 70.* put one arm round the patient's shoulders and one under their thighs. As the patient leans back, lift the legs as you support the body.

KEEP CLOSE, KEEP SUPPLE !

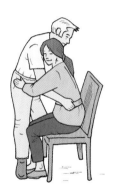
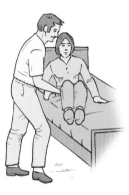

TRANSPORT

By Car:

- You are running late, you dash to the garage, your smart sports car is waiting for you. Its very low and sleek ! You jump in, you are practically lying down, legs and arms stretched to their limits as you speed onto the motorway. Ah ! Huge traffic jam. You are furious, clench your teeth and tense your arms and hands on the wheel. You arrive at work 20 minutes late, leap out of the car, sprint to the office, your neck and shoulders are stiff, your head hurts and your lower back kills you all day long !

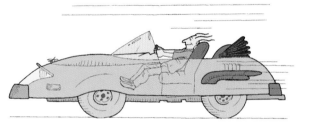

- You've anticipated there will be a traffic jam this morning, so you are 15 minutes early when leaving the house. You have realised that bad backs and sports cars don't go together so you have a nice car in the garage, but it has an adjustable seat which tilts up-down, a good supportive back rest with an adjustable bump at the lower back level. Your steering wheel has a height adjustment.

- You sit on the car seat, arm/hands holding the door frame or steering wheel. You move legs, hips, bottom, and shoulders all together until you are sitting comfortably and you repeat the movement to get out of the car. Your seat should be adjusted forward so that your knees are bent when your feet touch the pedals. Tilt your seat so that the whole of your thigh is in contact with the seat. Your elbows should be slightly bent, adjust the steering wheel or use a firm back support cushion or lumbar roll so that your back is straight and totally supported. The head rest should support your head, not your neck for security reasons. You arrive on time and you feel fine !

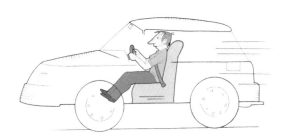

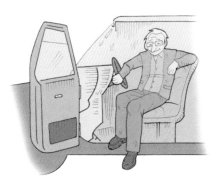

Packing the Car and Long Journeys

- Try to choose a car with an easy flat access to
  the boot or trunk. Avoid cars with a raised rim
  where you need to lift articles over it.
  Sometimes if you have large objects, think of
  loading into the back seat of the car. Lean
  with hands/arms/body wherever you can.
  Use the Pelvic Tilt ⚠ exercise, tightening
  buttocks and tummy muscles as you lift. Lean
  against the bumper or put one knee on the back
  seat of the car. Put heaviest objects close to
  the edge of the boot so its easier to remove
  them. If you have packages on the front passenger seat, get out of the car and go round to
  remove them, instead of stretching from the
  driver's seat. Avoid twisting when you need to
  look behind, move your hips, stretch one arm on
  to the back of the passenger seat, use your
  mirrors. On long journeys, stop for 10 minutes
  every two hours, get out of the car, move, walk
  and stretch !

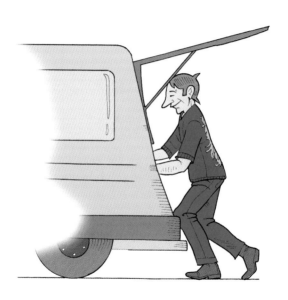

Driving Lorries, Vans and Agricultural Machinery

- Use the same rules as those for driving a car. Add to that the importance of a good seat which absorbs shocks. Most modern lorries and tractors are fitted with these seats, check that yours is well maintained. If you find yourself on bumpy or hard surfaces, try to sit on the edge of the seat and keep buttocks clenched tight to protect your vertebrae against unnecessary shocks. Lift yourself off the seat slightly, holding on to the steering wheel if you are on very difficult terrain. Stop, stand up, walk about and stretch at frequent intervals.

KEEP CLOSE, KEEP STRAIGHT, KEEP SUPPLE !

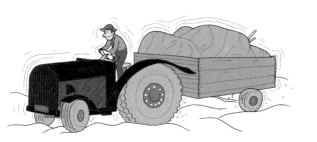

Travelling by Plane

- There is no worse form of transport for your back than travelling by plane, but few people can do without them these days ! The seats have been designed to insure security rather than comfort, and you may be often cramped in the sitting position for hours whilst your neighbour snores away under his eyeshade and blanket with your only escape being to climb over him !

- Inform your airline in advance if you are a back sufferer. Very often they can arrange for a seat on the aisle or with extra leg room, and in severe cases can sometimes allow you two seats to lie down. As soon as it's possible, recline your seat, experiment with a blow up cushion for your neck, use the airline cushion in your neck, upper or lower back, or bring your own lumbar roll which can help to fill in the gaps in airline seats. Protect your neck with a scarf if the air conditioning is too cold. Use the foot rest bar if you have one, or rest your knees briefly on the seat in front. Do some of the stretching exercises for sitting that you'll find on *page 166-167*. Get up and walk the aisles as much and as often as you can. Remember to drink plenty of water to prevent dehydration.

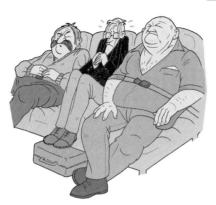

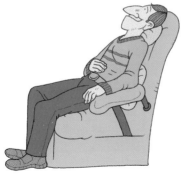

Luggage

- Whether you travel by train, boat or plane, it is rare that you can avoid having to lift or heave baggage at some point or other.

- Pack wisely. If you know you will be on your own, limit your baggage. Choose two small soft bags rather than one huge rigid one. Test them before purchasing that they may run well on wheels, that you can push as well as pull the case and that you are not bent double when you do so. Try to push your bags, but if you have to pull - keep your arms tucked into your side with the bags as close to you as possible. Remember that your hand luggage should be as light as possible. These bags are often the ones you will have to put on high shelves or lift on and off security rolling carpets. Use a shoulder bag with a strap that you can wear diagonally or a back pack with pockets that open on the inside for security reasons.

- Travelling with a large back pack - make sure the straps are adjusted for you. Your pack should be as high as possible on your back. Use the waist strap to relieve pressure on neck and shoulders. Avoid rigid packs and top heavy packing.

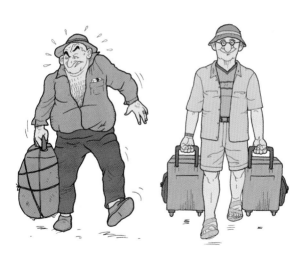

SPORT AND LEISURE

Introduction:

- There is nothing better for your mind or body than to have a change of routine and to participate in a sport or leisure activity that gives you PLEASURE ! Because you may have a bad back it does not mean you cannot participate in sporting activities, on the contrary depriving yourself of something you enjoy will only make you more depressed which may increase your back pain.

But there are important points to bear in mind:

- Talk to your doctor or therapist about recommencing. Start off slowly, train progressively. Start for short periods building up slowly. Note how you feel the following day.
- If your back pain is worse, stop and restart a week later.

- Always shower or bath immediately after an activity that makes you perspire. Change damp clothes. Use a towel around your neck and shoulders. Avoid draughts. Make sure your shoes are adapted for the activity.

Before participating in any sport, some stretching exercises standing or sitting *page 166-169*, will ensure that during or after the activity you will suffer less back pain.

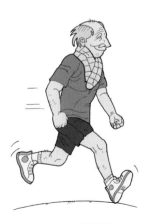

Recommended **Sports**

Are those:
- That give you pleasure.
- That use several groups of muscles.
- That enable harmonious sequence of movements.
- That help your balance.
- That stimulate your heart and circulation and help your endurance.
- That do not require rapid extremes of effort.
- That do not involve hard shocks to the back.

- *Walking:* Use a good pair of walking shoes or sports shoes, walk on soft ground - the grass verge, in woods, on sand. Avoid hard or bumpy roads. Swing your arms, no hands in pockets. Stride, don't dawdle. Use the pelvic tilt exercise if you get tired.

- *Cross country skiing:* or the equivalent on an exercise machine. Excellent for your back if you use arms and legs correctly. It's harmonious, balanced (usually, except if you fall !), uses many groups of muscles and stimulates the heart.

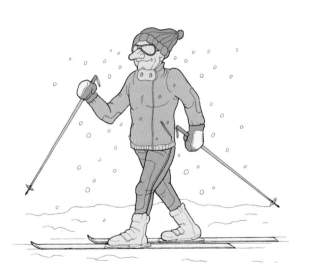

- *Gym and Stretching*: A combination of cardio-vascular workout on a soft surface with no jogging on the spot, and stretching exercises which progressively stretch your muscles: excellent for your back. Choose a gym and a teacher who have had proper training. If in doubt speak with your physiotherapist who will advise you.

- *Swimming:* Warm up by swimming on your back, or on your side (both directions). The crawl is fine as long as your back is straight, head in the water.
    - Avoid breast stroke unless you put your head in the water.
    - Avoid the butterfly and racing dives.

- *Cycling:* is good as long as your bicycle saddle, handlebars and frame have been adjusted for you personally. Make sure your knees and arms are still slightly flexed in the extreme positions.
    - Avoid mountain biking on hard ground.

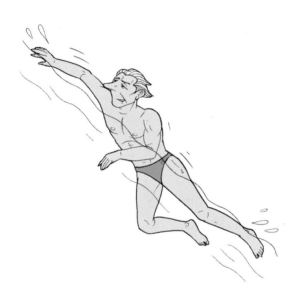

- *Tennis, badminton, squash, table tennis, basketball etc:* These are all activities which use one side of the body more than the other. Bilateral stretching exercises before playing will help to avoid back pain. Avoid playing on hard courts and surfaces. Warm up using the left hand if you are right handed and vice versa.

- *Golf:* Another sport which activates one side of the body more than the other. Stretching is essential before playing. Start with a half swing - left to right, and right to left, and always start your practice with chips and pitches on grass rather than mats. Try to walk on grass instead of hard paths, push your trolley, don't pull. Keep it close to your body, arms always bent. Use soft spikes - THINK SUPPLE ! *Pos 3 or 7 page 70-71* for picking up your ball.

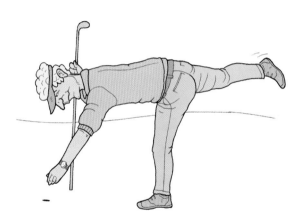

- *Football (soccer), downhill skiing, horse riding:* Are all recommended as long as you have trained, stretched and worked on lower body muscles and that you already possess a reasonable technique.

- *Jogging:* Only with training, good cushion soles in your shoes and on soft ground.
  - Jogging on roads and pavements can irritate and inflame a potential back problem.

- *Rowing:* Be prudent. A good technique is vital, otherwise it can cause lower back pain strain.

- *Pool, snooker, billiards:* Lean on the table, use thigh muscles to take the strain and keep your back straight.

Ask your physiotherapist about sports that may not be listed here.

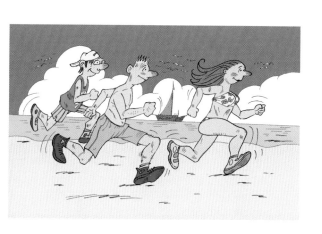

Sports Not Recommended

- *Water sports:* windsurfing, waterskiing etc. - because of the strain it can cause to the lower back.

- *Impact sports:* parachuting, hand gliding etc.

- *Trampoline:* particularly for children.

- *Violent sports:* rugby, American football, boxing etc.

Please remember that this is a guideline only. If you find in this list a sport you love, ask for medical or other appropriate professional advice about recommencing or continuing after back trouble.

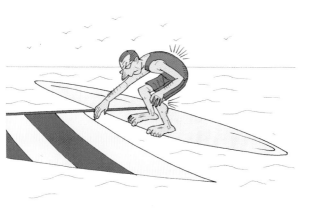

Leisure Activities

- Leisure activities are an extremely important part of helping to maintain our well being. Whatever you choose as a hobby is good for you. Make sure that if you are sitting for long periods, to re-read the sitting section of this book. The same applies if you are standing for long periods. Try to choose something that:

> **keeps you moving !**
> **keeps you supple !**
> **keeps you straight !**
> **keeps you close !**

A Word about Gardening

- Rather than giving up gardening because your back hurts, try to adjust your positions and if necessary change your materials to make you more comfortable.
- Use a pair of knee pads, this enables you to move around work on one knee, both knees or all fours.

- Change your position regularly, have frequent breaks.
- Use *positions 2/5/6/7 page 70-71*.
- Stop and make a pelvic tilt exercise before you feel pain coming on.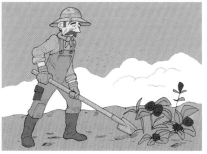
- Use long handled tools.

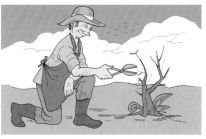

Stretching and Relaxation for the Whole Family

 • To be able to stretch correctly and to have the ability to relax will go a long way to helping you maintain a healthy mind, back and body. However, you should ask your physiotherapist for a personalised exercise or treatment programme when you have been recommended to do so by your doctor.

• Be realistic. Doing 5-10 minutes of stretching per day either **after** your shower in the morning or in the evening is much better for you than doing 40 minutes every day for a week and then doing nothing for a month.

• Choose a quiet time and a quiet place, if possible, turn off bright lights, use an exercise mat, play some relaxing music.

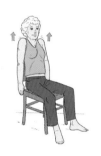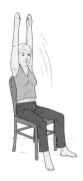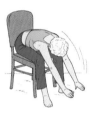

Sitting and Stretching

To be used either at the office, at your desk or at home.

- On a straight backed chair with no arm rest, feel relaxed, but try to make sure that during these exercises, your back (at waist or belt level) touches the back of the chair
  We tend to ignore the fact that a lot of tension can build up in our heads and neck, so always start with these simple stretching exercises for the head. All exercises should be performed slowly. Hold the stretch as long as possible, counting to between 6 and 10.

Hands behind head. Push head gently towards chest. Breathe in stretching up. Breathe out stretching down 3x.

①

Right hand to touch left ear and vice versa. Keep eyes and head horizontal. Stretch neck gently. 3x in each direction.

②

Gentle stretching circles with head twice in each direction. Arms relaxed by your side.

③

Breathe in. Lift one shoulder as high as possible keeping back straight and well stretched. Gently release breathing out at same time. 3x each shoulder

④

Breathe in. Lift both shoulders at the same time. Slowly release breathing out. 3x.

⑤

⑥

Stretch back, arms to ceiling, hands, fingers outspread. Breathe in, hold the stretch. Gently release, breathe out round back. Head between knees, arms flop, not necessarily to floor.
Very important : To come up. Tighten abdominal muscles and bottom, unroll one vertebra after the other to sitting position. 3x.

⑦

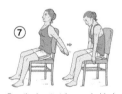

Breathe in, stretch arms behind chair. Hands together, stretch arms out behind at same time, push back (waist level) to back of the chair. Hold the stretch. Head not too far back. Breathe out. Head onto chest. Release arms.

⑧

Extend one leg at a time from sitting position. Flex and extend ankle, circles in both directions with each foot.

Standing, Lying and Stretching

 Exercises to do at home, after a shower or in the evening and before and after strenuous exercise.

 • Avoid doing these stretching exercises immediately after getting out of bed. Shower first !

①

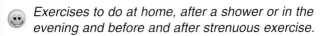

Stretch whole back and arms to ceiling. Breathe in. Hands, fingers outstretched.
Very important : Knees bent. Breathe out slowly. Round back. Push knees forward. Let head and arms flop towards floor. Feel back rounded and relaxing.

②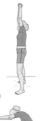

Very important : To come up. Push hips forward. Keep knees bent. Tighten abdominal muscles and bottom, unroll one vertebra after the other. 3x.

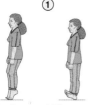

Standing on mat. Rise as high as possible on your toes. Fix a point and hold it. Roll back on to heels and lift toes off mat. 3x.

Kneel down. Sit on heels. Try to keep your bottom on your heels. Stretch arms as far as forward on mat as possible. Breathe in, hold stretch. Release arms, head, round back. Breathe out.

Sit on mat. Soles of feet facing each other. Hands holding ankles. Breathe in. Stretch the back. Look in front of you. Breathe out. Let back round. Head on chest.

 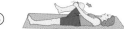

Lying on back. Head on mat. Make a double chin to stretch cervical vertebrae. Bring one knee up to chest, hold with arms. Look at your knee keeping head on mat. Breathe in. Hold. Breathe out. Release. 3x each leg.

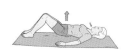

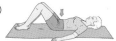

Lying on mat. Knees bent, arms by your side. Lift hips off mat. Hold, Flatten back against mat, pushing at waist height. 10x.

Lying on mat. Knees bent. Shoulders against mat. Roll knees from one side to the other. 3x

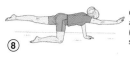

On all fours. Keeping back straight, tighten abdominals and buttocks. Stretch out left leg (no higher than horizontal) and right arm at same time. Reverse the procedure.

Stretching for Neck and Upper Back

Between the shoulder blades is a difficult area to exercise, and this is often where we have pain, if we sit, study and carry a lot. Try these three stretching exercises.

Stand against a wall. Knees bent with back pressed against the wall. Tighten buttocks and abdominal muscles. Shoulders against wall. Lift both arms at a right angle keeping them against the wall.

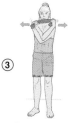

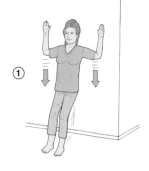

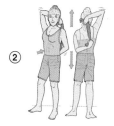

Standing with knees bent. Cross your arms behind your back. Don't arch your back. Using an old stocking one end in each hand, make 10 small stretches. Change arms and repeat.

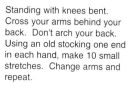

Standing with knees bent, arms crossed at elbows, in front of you away from chest. Using the old stockings, make 10 small stretches. Change arms and repeat.

Stretching to *Avoid*

These following exercises can aggravate your problem.

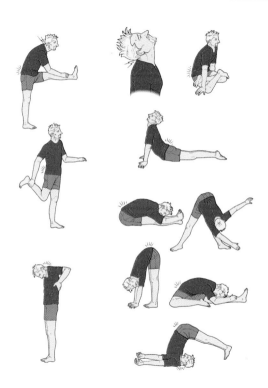

Relaxation Exercises

 • These movements are designed to help relax muscles that are tight and stressed. Choose a quiet place with no phones !
If you manage to do the whole of the stretching programme this is a good way to finish it off, otherwise these relaxation techniques can be used separately at any time if you feel stressed or even in bed if you can't sleep.

• Stretch out on the floor or on your bed. With eyes closed and arms by your side, breathe at your own rhythm slowly and deeply.

• Tighten all the muscles of your face, your eyes, ears and your skull, slowly release the muscles breathing out deeply.

• Tighten your neck, chest, shoulders and arms down to your hands and fingers. Hold your breath, release, breathe out.

- Tighten the muscles of your back, chest, stomach, hips and buttocks. Hold your breath, release, breathe out.

- Tighten your buttocks, your hips, thighs, knees, calves, ankles, feet and toes. Hold your breath, release and breathe out.

- Tighten up your whole body from head to toe, release slowly breathe out.

- Bend your knees, make three deep breathing exercises. Breathe in filling your diaphragm and lungs with air, breathe out, squeezing the air out of your diaphragm and lungs.

- Lie still for two minutes breathing normally.

- Roll on to your side, then on to all fours, standing up from this position.

Conclusion

I have aimed in this little book to give a few simple, practical explanations of how best to understand your back and why it might be hurting. The solutions need your active participation. There are no easy ways out. You are solely responsible for trying to make the activities in your daily life more comfortable. I hope that if you can read this book, and maybe laugh a little, perhaps recognising yourself in some of these scenarios, that you can also realise how far a positive attitude can go towards helping your problem.

Look back at page 12. Is your piece of paper still on the fridge door ? Have you done something about what causes you stress in your life ?

Should you think of nothing else after reading these lines, **please**:

THINK STRAIGHT !
THINK CLOSE !
THINK SUPPLE !
And KEEP MOVING !